*Don't Stop Short of the Blessing:
My Journey to Weight Loss*

Don't Stop Short of the Blessing:
My Journey to Weight Loss

Kendra A. Wood, Ed.D.

Dedication

This book is to my best friends Dinecia and She' Nita who have supported me and given me grace on this journey. This book is also for my brother Keith. You motivated me to take my first real steps. I hope this book motivates you as you restart your journey! We got this for life!

Contents

It all started with a pound and a prayer...

1.61 Pounds Down

July 2, 2019

Lord,

I believe you will fulfill your promise to be strong where I am weak, that you would be with me wherever I go. I am on a journey to weight loss. As I was walking today, the thought came to me to use this journal to log my fitness activity every day. Today I walked the neighborhood for 22 minutes. The last time I stepped on the scale was Friday June 28. I weighed in at 285.9 pounds. I was down 1.6 pounds since June 1. This was after four days of dieting. I am on vacation this week, so I won't fully be back on the diet until next Monday. I will try not to go too overboard. I would like to be down by 30-60 pounds by January.

Amen

This was a journal entry not too long after I completed my doctoral journey. A few years prior to this I made an agreement with my primary care doctor that I would finish my doctorate and then lose the weight. This agreement was made after failed attempts of losing weight over a few months and after a diagnosis of hypertension.

I never did write in that journal about my weight loss again. In fact, it turned out to be a pray for my husband journal. That's a whole different book for me to write in another season, whenever I do get that husband!

So here I am now picking up where I left off in hopes to document my weight loss journey. I also hope to share encouragement with some other person that might need a little extra motivation to make it happen.

16 Pounds Down

October 2020

I am 16 pounds down. I have had so many false starts over the years. My prayer to the Lord at 1.61 pounds down in my journal is a testament to this. I can look back in my Facebook and Instagram memories and it was usually late summer, early fall. I'd see posts of me exercising, a salad, or a green smoothie, with a caption, "I am really sticking to it this time". Each time I didn't. I found myself starting over again the next year that time.

New Year's Day 2020, I showed up at a family function. I knew my brother Keith had been doing a little working out but to my surprise he had dropped 40 pounds. For the first time in probably ever, he was smaller than me or at least on his way. We took pictures and the pictures screamed that I had reached my limit. I remember feeling a bit jealous and a whole lot of disappointment that I had gained so much weight.

A few months later the pandemic hit, and I thought hey, here's my chance. I will swap my drive time for exercise. My mom and I started daily walks at 4:30pm each day after I got off from working remotely. Those walks were hard. I could barely make it to 30 minutes. There was this sneaky hill in my neighborhood that I dreaded every single walk. I would get frustrated. How is my almost 70-year-old mother leaving me in the dust? A month or so went by. I think I may have dropped almost eight pounds. The progress seemed slow. I still ate ice cream and pizza and the things that counter acted my walking.

However, the walks became easier. I was getting closer to a 30 minute walk each day. One of the motivating factors for those walks was my ability to walk past the house I was building. Each day my mom and I got to see the progress and speculate what would come next.

In May, I closed on my house and moved in. The move exhausted me. Had it not been for my brother, younger cousin, his friend, an aunt, and uncle along with my mom, I do not know how I would have made that move happen. After the unpacking, the walks stopped and I had my full enjoyment of new house, cookies, cake, ice cream, wine, and more.

Then the end of July came. The end of July came in with the breath of fresh air I needed, a new job! For those who do not know, I began job searching a year or so before I completed my doctorate. My close friends and family knew that this was a part of my life that was weighing heavy on me. I was burned out in the worst way! Because of my burnout, I found comfort in stress and emotional eating. While I know my career, field is where I am supposed to be, the frontline role at a small institution just takes something out of you.

With my new job and breath of fresh air I was able to re-evaluate my eating habits and level of physical activity. I was able to get more active and had the mental capacity and determination to start my weight loss journey. Stress is a huge factor in weight loss. The presence of it makes it hard to lose weight. The absence of it makes it hard not to lose weight with the right diet and exercise.

So, here I am, early October 2020 16 pounds down. My goal is to lose 50 pounds by my birthday in January 2021 and focus on losing another 50 pounds in the remainder of 2021.

I saw a post that talked about how when people post before and after pictures, they often get comment's like "That can't be the same person." The post went on to say, "Do you expect them to be the same person?" This really got me to thinking, that no, those people are not the same person. They have gone through a transformation, not just physically but emotionally, mentally, and often spiritually.

I intend to come out of this a different person. I hope that my process involves pinpointing my triggers, understanding why I had such an unhealthy relationship with food, and how I can live a healthier life. So, what do I know about myself and my relationship with food?

Emotional Eater and Sleeper

One thing I know for sure is that I am an emotional eater. The day my dad died, I had to drive from North Carolina to Virginia to see him one last time. On my way to see him I stopped at Chick-fil-A and got a peach milkshake. I could only imagine how I would feel if he had passed away before I got there. God's grace was sufficient in not letting that be an emotional scar for me. I made it there to say goodbye even with a stop for a peach milkshake.

My drug of choice for my hurt, pain, grief, and stress has always been food by way of some sugary sweet dessert. Ask any of my family and they'll confirm that I make the best pound cake, sweet potato pie, and banana pudding. Ask my former coworkers and they'll tell you they miss mini-Bundt rum cakes at Christmas.

I prefer my own homemade desserts over other people's desserts. One year I wanted to buy a birthday cake for my mom. After several tastings of bakeries and stores, I opted for a cheesecake factory cheesecake because all the regular cakes I came across were dry! They were nothing in comparison to my cakes and I could not bring myself to buy a dry cake! It would not be acceptable for me or my family!

It was nothing for me to get in a mood and bake a pound or rum cake to try and make myself feel better. When it comes to my emotional eating, one of the other things I noticed was that when it all seemed to weigh on me heavy, I opted to take a nap.

Now a nap and a snack are biblical. We know that from the story of Elijah in 1 Kings 19. Elijah was at the point where he was so overwhelmed with what was going on in his life that he prayed for God to let him die! God answers his prayer by allowing him to sleep, eat, and sleep again!

Sometimes biblical even gets taken out of context. There was purpose behind Elijah's eating and sleeping and that was so that he could get up and make the rest of his

17

forty-day and forty-night journey! When life has us overwhelmed and stuck, we can't eat and sleep and stay in the same place! We must fuel up to keep going toward our purpose!

Context is important! As I think about context, I must reflect on how in the Black community food is love. Food is comfort. Food is community. Food is safety. Growing up, I could not go to my grandma Irma's house without her asking me five times if I was hungry. If I obliged on the first ask, I would get two maybe even three asks if I had enough or wanted more. I am quite sure other Black people have had this same experience and can tell you that they were conditioned to just be ready to eat when they went to see their grandma.

One comfort food I can remember was Grandma Irma's homemade applesauce from the apples on the apple tree in her yard. Of course, there were other favorites like fried oysters, pork chops, chicken, or a special treat from the Schwan's truck. But in that space, in that context, my belly was always full, and I knew I was loved.

I also looked at my grandma in her last days in her battle with cancer. My aunt tried hiding a pack of chocolate chip cookies from her because they did not want her to eat too many. Grandma Irma found those cookies and enjoyed them! I thought about that and in my mind, if Grandma Irma could live a full life into her eighties, eating exactly what she wanted, then why not me? Now why not me is because Grandma Irma was born in 1927 and grew up on real food. Me on the other hand, I was an 80s baby, and right in the middle of the processed food era.

My favorite holiday has always been Thanksgiving. I generally spent my Thanksgivings growing up with my mom's side of the family, the Burgesses. I can remember that one Thanksgiving, I ate until I made myself sick. So much pie, pound cake, greens, sweet potato pie, mac and cheese, Aunt Corene's rolls, yams until I found myself throwing up in my grandma Dof's bathroom. The food and the time were again, love, comfort, and security. Knowing that all my family was around, eating to my heart's content was what made me happy, even if temporary.

Maybe Thanksgiving with the Burgesses was such a big deal because it gave me the joy, that was lost when my nuclear family was broken apart. My parents divorced when I was in the second grade. My mom, brother, and I packed it up and moved to North Carolina. Maybe Thanksgiving with the Burgesses also represented the one time in the year that we had such an abundance of food and no worries. Far from the ramen noodle struggle days of Sulfur Spring Road in Warrenton.

Work Life

I think most millennials have a story about being miserable in a job. I think for me, after graduating from college, I kept finding myself in the role of a frontline worker, the catch all type worker. This goes for the non-profit, education, and other jobs held. I seemed to get all the inquiries and problems everyone else didn't know how to solve or want to deal with. Being the front line will burn you out. Being the front line will also make you pack on the pounds. I mean think about it, 40 hours a week, at a computer and desk. From 2011-2019 I gained at least fifty pounds if not more.

Dear college graduates, there is this thing called the "Adulting 50" if you are not careful! If you have failed to lose your freshman 15-40, you are really in trouble! Please make sure that just as hard as you are working to make a name for yourself in your career, you are also taking care of your physical, mental, spiritual, and emotional self.

Jobs and even careers come and go but what you don't want to go is YOU!

Maybe I was depressed in my work life. I'm sure I was depressed in general. Well, I know for sure, I developed a vitamin d deficiency. As I think back, I had maybe a year that my thoughts were so cloudy that I couldn't concentrate. The fluorescent lights and computer screens bothered my eyes. I was just tired. No matter what I did, I couldn't get enough rest or clear my mind.

Doctoral Days

Maybe it was that thing that happens to you when you work on your doctorate. You know they say that you go a little crazy when you complete your doctorate. While I was in it, I denied the crazy part. I prided myself on not going crazy while completing that degree. But maybe I did. One thing I am learning about myself, especially as I learn about trauma and how to treat people when they've gone through something is that you can't base a person's trauma on the level of how they react to the trauma. Some people will look at someone who is not screaming and crying about a traumatic event and say that they must be lying because it is not the expected reaction.

As with me, I am calm and even keel always. I rarely get worked up. So, while I may have been depressed and freaking out inside over my doctoral journey, from the outside you couldn't tell. At least in my actions. I think about the meme that says, "Ya'll sat around and watched me get fat. Ya'll are not my true friends!" That was the sign! So, for future reference if ya'll see me getting fat again, check on me! I may not be okay!

Although I didn't get all worked up over my doctoral journey, I did gain weight. I made myself the promise that once I completed my doctorate, I would lose this weight. An entire year later and the weight is still here. But not for long.

47.2 Pounds Down!

January 5, 2021

A few days ago, I tried on a dress I bought in 2016 for a cruise to Bermuda. I can remember putting on girdle. I may have even put on my best friend Dinecia's girdle on top of my girdle and sucked it in so that she could struggle to zip the dress up for the captain's ball. I have been trying on this dress for maybe a month now and I was able to put it on and zip it up without a girdle on! The non-scale victories are just as rewarding as the scale victories!

As I reflect on my fitting in to that dress it just dawned on me how much I have tried to fit in to spaces that I don't fit! For one reason or another at those times, I did not fit and now I am realizing that is ok. I am finding that in just the right time, I am fitting in to the clothes and spaces that God wants me to. I can't rush to fit. You can't either!

So far, I am about five months in to consistently being on this journey. I've learned that it is about a mindset and a commitment. I also learned that I've been doing a whole lot of eating out of boredom or emotion. Now, however, I am eating out of necessity, and I am even exercising out of desire!

I make it a habit to move every day. If I find that most of the day has gone by and I have not hit my Fitbit steps for the day, I pop on a YouTube walking video and get to stepping! I generally have to push myself to do morning workouts which I know will burn more fat since I am in the fasted state.

A good sweat helps me feel better throughout the day. I am not sure if a chapter or so from now I will be telling you that I have kicked up my workouts and am doing some crazy killer workouts but as of right now, at 47.2 pounds down, my bread-and-butter workouts have been walking! With simply counting calories and walking I am nearly halfway to my weight goal!

Did I mention I am struggling with buying clothes? I am a shopper! I cannot help it. I thought I had made my mind up to not buy clothes until I lost a significant amount of weight. Well, I lied to myself, and I am paying for it now. I am realizing that I am so used to my larger dress sizes that I am buying my clothes too big. I am out here second guessing myself! I went to Walmart the other day and bought a cute sweater. I initially picked up a size 16-18 so confidently but then went back and switched it out for a 20.

Why did I do that? The sweater is too big! From now on I will trust myself to size down or not buy at all. I have to train my eye again. In my psyche I am still a larger size but in my physical it is coming on down.

I have about four size 18 pairs of jeans that I can put on, zip, and button but not actually wear yet. I pray that by my birthday January 27 or Valentine's Day, I can wear those jeans. I mean, I really do not have anywhere to go due to the pandemic, but the pictures would look nice!

53.2 Pounds Down

January 21, 2021

I thought I would start the next chapter with some flowery birthday message about how I've hit or exceeded my birthday weight loss goal (which I have), but I am a week ahead of my birthday and need to address the concept of eating what your momma cooked/put on the table.

We often scoff at how the kids these days are just too picky in their eating and say, "When I was growing up, I ate what my momma cooked!" It often surprises me how picky these kids are. I am also often intrigued by the allergies the younger generations have. I have absolutely no allergies and growing up, everything my momma put on the table for me, I ate. My momma never had to force feed me or sneak in veggies. I ate what she cooked, and it was good. I have always lived by the concept of eating what was cooked for me.

However, today highlights just how difficult it is to be conscious about my eating and weight loss journey when living with someone. For me, yes, it is my momma. My momma lives with me. I have my own personal chef, ya'll! No, I appreciate the fact that she cooks and free's me to chase my career!

This week, I have been trying to cut my carbs and have been seeing results with almost four pounds lost. I even mentioned to my momma about my incorporation of a keto lunch option instead of my usual salad. I'm upstairs and suddenly I smell beans. Beans wouldn't be so bad if I perhaps didn't have my carb packed smoothie this morning which came in a whopping 47 grams of carbs.

A cup of beans also comes in at 47 grams of carbs. In addition to the beans, when I came downstairs, I discovered a box of Jiffy cornbread sitting on the counter to be baked. Cornbread comes in at around 37 grams of carbs. My only bright light was the ground turkey thawing. Ok, maybe I could eat a turkey burger and make veggies and forgo the beans and cornbread.

Nope! Momma proceeds to cook the ground turkey and add it to the beans! So, at the earliest, I may be able to eat what my momma cooked tomorrow. If I skip the smoothie for breakfast, keep my low carb lunch, and then have the beans for dinner.

This not only sheds light on the struggle of healthy eating when living with others but also the engrained habits and beliefs around eating. I've gone so many years eating to not offend someone. You show at someone's house, and they offer you food, so you eat. Or, a coworker brings breakfast casserole or cheesecake, so you eat!

I also spent years eating so the other person would not eat alone. I remember when one of my friends was living with me. I would have eaten my dinner. He would come in from work. Look at what I cooked. Eat it or not, and then ask can you order a pizza?

I would order pizza and eat pizza with him! He often teases me because I called the pizza place one day and when they answered they were like "ok and is this, Kendra Wood?" We have technology to thank for them knowing who I was. You know, phone numbers, the Dominoes app. It really was my friend's fault that I ordered that much pizza in that season in my life, whether he wants to admit to it or not!

Today I'm learning the lesson that it's ok not to eat the beans. It's ok not to eat the pizza. I am also learning that I am the only one that can track and control my weight loss journey, no matter who's doing the cooking.

55.4 Pounds Down

February 8, 2021

Yesterday I weighed in at 227.6 pounds. That put me at 55.4 pounds down. I finally dropped another pound and a half since my birthday. I must admit, last week was my first week back on track since my birthday and this week will be off again. Today is my momma's birthday! Happy Birthday momma! She is 69 years young.

It is also Valentine's week of which I hope to get some sort of chocolate. My church is having a Mardi Gras drive through celebration of which I plan on ordering a plate and enjoying some good old bread pudding. Today I have already indulged in seafood pasta salad, German chocolate cake, and vanilla ice cream.

We zoomed right past my birthday of which I need to revisit. Upon the announcement of my 53-pound weight loss I was sprinkled with an array of inboxes from people asking what I did to lose the weight. By the evening of my birthday, I had drafted a prewritten statement and would make edits, if necessary, based on the questions they asked. Note to self, have this book all wrapped up and ready to order when you make the 100-pound weight loss announcement!

So, what did I do to lose 53 pounds?

Exercise

I mainly just walked 30 minutes or more 3-5 times a week. When it was warm outside, my mom and I would walk the neighborhood. Since it has gotten cold outside, I've turned to YouTube. I usually get up every morning and put on one of Rick Buehler's walking videos. His 5000-step video is generally my default but if I oversleep then I do a shorter video and make sure I go with my mom when she walks my dog Lennox twice a day. He's really her dog now. He sticks really close to her since her dog Coco passed away.

Earlier in my journey I also had fun doing KuKuwa fitness videos on YouTube. Back in middle and high school I was a part of a mentoring group called "The Whole Village." I went through a rites of passage program and one of the main components of the program was African dance. From that experience I have a love for African dance and can actually say that timeframe in life was the one other time I lost weight and kept it off. I was excited when I found the KuKuwa fitness YouTube page, but I got a little ahead of myself because I messed my foot and ankle up real quick. I was down with that injury for like three weeks. I do plan on trying it again now that I have dropped such a significant amount of weight.

Diet

In terms of my eating, I cut out sweets, breads, sodas, and refined carbs. Mainly I cut out junk and ate clean. I ate about 1200-1300 calories a day. At first it was hard but now I don't find myself hungry. That is a super low number of calories and probably not sustainable so you would just need to find what works for you. I know that this worked for me as a tool along the journey to get the weight off. There are a bunch of calorie calculators out there that can help with finding this balance.

There are some weeks that my calorie intake inches up to 1400-1500 calories and that generally works out as well because with my exercise I usually end up below my calorie intake for the day. I used my Fitbit to set my calorie goals and set it so that my goal was to have a 1000 calorie deficit a day. With this deficit the average weight loss a week is two pounds.

I drink plenty of water. When I say drink plenty of water, I mean half my body weight in ounces of water! I kept reading online where these women say that they drink a gallon of water a day and it dawned on me, girl you're drinking a little over a gallon a day!

My saving grace in this season has been that I am working remotely. I can pee in peace without feeling judged. I can also poop two, three, four, or five times in peace as well! So that reminds me that in addition to water, I drink a detox tea. Find a detox tea that works for you and keep it on deck.

I generally drink about 16 ounces of detox tea a day. I count those ounces toward my fluid intake and generally either drink the tea straight or with some lemon. Some days I drink the tea hot and other days I drink it cold. I also often put my morning dose of tea in my smoothie instead of using water or some type of milk. It keeps me regular for sure!

To be more specific about my eating, I eat a lot of the same foods honestly. I either have baked fish or baked chicken with veggies. I eat fried fish as well. That is about the only fried thing I eat. I eat turkey burgers, steamed mixed or one type of veggies. I do a lot of stir fries. Kroger has this fresh stir fry veggie kit that I usually have with shrimp or chicken.

I do cauliflower rice instead a regular rice. I noticed early on that rice, even brown rice, was not my friend and I would need to avoid it. I also found this to be true with sweet potatoes which I had all intentions of using as a substitute for white potatoes.

I generally eat two boiled eggs in the morning with a smoothie (berries, lemon, beets, ginger, turmeric, spinach banana, apples, avocado... whatever I have lol), coffee and Nutpods creamer which is plant based and only 10 calories a tablespoon. Lunch is usually a salad, some keto combo I have come up with, or a personal cauliflower crust pizza. Yes, I know I said keto does not work for me. That does not mean I can't have a keto meal here or there. Dinners are usually where the turkey burgers, chicken, and stir fry meals come in.

The other thing I have started exploring is plant-based meat substitutes. Meatless Monday needed something so I wouldn't starve so I started out with a plant-based brat to go in stir fry veggies. I have also tried out meatless chicken nuggets and can proudly say I tried tofu in a stir fry, and it was not bad at all!

The reactions of my family and friends are funny. While they are often on board with the moderation of diet, when I start talking fake meat, they are like oh no! They are not sold but here's my thing, I am going to eat what I want! So that means if I want plant-based sausage today and steak tomorrow, so be it as long as it stays within my calories!

Keeping a Food Journal

Logging the food in my Fitbit has helped to track the calories and then it also helps to go back and see what I ate on weeks that I lost the most weight. Logging the food helps with keeping the right portion sizes. Logging the food also helps place a level of accountability for me. Granted, no one else sees my food logs but it is just a reminder to me that I need to stay within the healthy boundaries I have placed for myself.

While I no longer keep a food log, having the habit of logging my food added a layer of consciousness to my eating. Without logging my food, I can still judge whether I am overeating simply by being mindful of what I eat and how I feel when I eat.

Reading Food Labels

I do a lot of reading the label on the foods as well. My mind has been blown at how we eat well above and beyond the serving sizes on the labels. All my life I used to eat the whole bag of chips or six of the cookies when a serving size is a fourth of a bag of chips or two of the cookies. Portion and serving sizes are a real thing and they matter. I generally stick to the serving sizes on the food labels unless my calories have room to double a portion.

I also have this thing now where I am annoyed when I see a plate with a huge portion of meat and a small portion of veggies. Give me my veggies! While having high protein is great, why not have just as much if not more veggies on the plate than the meat?

Reading about Diet and Exercise

Whenever I think about certain aspects of my diet or changes, I want to make to my routine I google it. I read relevant articles and I watch a few YouTube videos. It is so important to be informed about the choices you make in your weight loss journey. Reading allows you to avoid the mistakes that others have already made. It also helps to build a feasible and sustainable action plan for the journey ahead.

For instance, I am exploring adding jogging into my exercise routine. My cousin She'Nita thinks that jogging helps to reduce belly fat because of the core muscles you have to use during the motion of jogging. This reminds me, I walked four miles on a Saturday in 20 something degrees in Northern Virginia with She'Nita!

I had just thought to myself how I would love to know whether I could ever to the Monument Avenue 10k again. She'Nita did not tell me the trail was 4 miles until we started walking. I freaked out a bit internally but once I hit mile one, I knew I could do it! We finished the trail in about an hour and twenty minutes and we also jogged for a short portion.

So, what am I watching YouTube videos about and reading up on now? Yes, you guessed it! How to start jogging. From one of the videos, I learned that one of the best ways to start jogging or running is to start off running 10-30 seconds at a time. Minimal yes but effective in getting started.

With that piece of knowledge, I have substituted a few intervals in my morning walk YouTube routine with jogging in place. I'll let you know whether it was feasible and sustainable to add jogging into my workout routine. I know what is most feasible and sustainable for my journey ahead is eating what I want! In moderation of course.

Eat what I want!

What I mean by this is that for my birthday week I ate crab cakes, cake, extra coffee, drank wine, and had chocolate covered strawberries, drank Northern Neck Ginger Ale, and cocktails. I enjoyed my birthday and yet I am 1.5 pounds lighter than my birthday weight. That is because I went back to my routine of eating healthy and exercising.

As I ate my German chocolate cake and ice cream with my momma today for her birthday, I thought to myself, this is why I was addicted to sweets! It was so good. Like really good to the point, I felt a little high! Perhaps it gave me a boost of endorphins or a sugar rush at the least! Will I continue to eat German chocolate cake every day? Absolutely not! There are two more pieces of German chocolate cake in the freezer for who knows how long. There is also vanilla ice cream in the freezer because the pint of Haagen das was only 40 cents less than whole gallon of ice cream. The adult in me just could not pay all that money for that little bit of ice cream.

While one of the things you may be saying to yourself is that is a lot. I do not want to do all of that. I didn't want to do it at one point either. You must get to a mental, even spiritual place of knowing and determination that you are ready to take on this journey. You may not choose to do the same things I did but, choose what works for you.

You know what does not work for me, keto! Keto, nor any other restrictive diet that has too many rules. I am a keep it simple kind of girl. I do not have the time for overcomplicated. That is why I drink my water, count my calories, understand what foods help and hinder my journey and find a balance.

60.7 Pounds Down

February 22, 2021

Today I weighed in at 222.2 pounds. I am still in awe of how this thing is really working for me! I am also in awe of the fact that I am only about 42 pounds from my goal weight of 180. When I was at the 20- and 40-pound marks I dreamt of the day that I would be over halfway to my goal. I am here!

I feel great. While I never will be a morning person, once I wake up and get my workout in, I feel energized! I have a clear mind and I am genuinely happy. I find myself praising God after a workout like yes! Thank you, Jesus! You have brought me a long way from depressed and physically uncomfortable from the weight. I mean, from my breathing, sciatica, heavy stomach, heart flutters, and low energy to now having none of those issues! I am utterly grateful. All it has taken is some persistence and some restraint.

That reminds me, my mom and I did not hold any restraint on that German Chocolate cake and ice cream. We ate the second piece the day after her birthday! The good news, however, was that it was now out of the house, and it did not hinder my progress. In fact, the remainder of that week did not hinder my progress either.

My church had a Mardi Gras celebration in which we had Mardi Gras Cajun pasta with shrimp, andouille sausage and chicken, green bean medley, salad, roll and bread pudding for dessert! I skipped lunch to stay within my calories and thoroughly enjoy the meal! I ate all my food and a few bites of the bread pudding. Having cut out sweets, the bread pudding was super sweet to my taste, so I had to wait a few days before I finished it.

In addition to Mardi Gras, Valentine's Day was in the mix as well. My best friend Dinecia sent me my favorite chocolates, Lindor Truffles, and of course in best friend fashion she sent me a pack of a whopping 75 truffles! She apologized for how they may hinder my journey. However, we made a plan of which I am sticking to. I ate a few and the rest are in my freezer!

It works out though. Those truffles are in my freezer which means I won't be tempted to buy any type of sugary sweet treat because I already have chocolates on hand. We'll see what lasts longer my truffles or my Northern Neck Ginger Ale that was discontinued and I'm keeping a stash of!

Even with all the sweets and atypical meals during my mom's birthday, Mardi Gras, and Valentine's Day week, my journey was not harmed. Those pairs of size 18 jeans that I mentioned, I was able to fit on Valentine's Day and wear! I can wear three out of the four pairs. The fourth pair, I think was a size 16 labeled as an 18 because they are just not happening! And it's ok! I rarely leave the house and I rarely wear jeans! The pandemic is still going strong and working remotely has allowed my new wardrobe to consist of tights and sweatshirts! I can transition from work to workout in seconds!

One of my goals that I have for this weight loss journey is to either come completely off or reduce my blood pressure and fluid pills. Since it is almost time to renew my prescription, I decided to schedule an appointment with my doctor to check in and see the possibility of this. I have an appointment on Wednesday of this week, and I am hopeful. My brother Keith was able to come off his diabetes medication after he lost a significant amount of weight. I want to be like him when I grow up! I will let you know how my appointment goes!

Well, I'm still on my blood pressure and fluid medications for now. I am going to put a heavy emphasis on the for now aspect of that sentence. In true fashion I went to my appointment, blood pressure logs from December up until now in tow and of course my blood pressure reading came in at 133/84. That was my lowest of several readings. It was probably my nerves, but I will take it as the Lord not saying no, but not yet.

The doctor mentioned that I could experiment with my fluid pills and let her know how it goes. I am just going to keep taking my meds as prescribed. She asked me if I had any symptoms of hypotension such as dizziness or any low blood pressure readings. I have not had any of those symptoms, but I now know what to look for.

I will go back in six months which also coincides with my annual checkup. By then my goal is to have dropped another forty if not more pounds. It is my hope that by then I will also have lowered my blood pressure and be at the point where I can come off those medications. I am in no way discouraged by today's visit to the doctor. I am well. My blood pressure is regulated with my medications, and I can't complain.

I also spoke with my doctor about the COVID-19 vaccine. I have not gotten it yet but because I am an educator, I can get on the priority list to get the vaccine. She gave me her take on the vaccine and her experiences. She had some mild side effects but nothing too severe.

She let me know that when I get the second dose, make plans to have some down time for the next few days as I could get flu like symptoms. But she explained that it makes sense because your body must build up some sort of immunity. I plan on at least signing up for the vaccine waitlist and we will see when I get it.

61.8 Pounds Down

March 3, 2021

I've been holding steady at the 61.8 pounds down for about a week and haven't had much to document on my journey until today. I would like to break out of the 220's but I know this is a marathon and not a sprint. However, I did have such a gratifying non-scale victory today. I really have to stop giving Old Navy all my money. I went shopping for gifts at Old Navy during Christmas time and have not been able to stop ordering stuff since.

My workout wardrobe has been graced with $12 and $10 Old Navy tights and sports bras. You know, companies have caught on to the whole weight loss, workout gear movement and are selling tights for $50 or more. Gone are the days that you could simply go grab a few pair of workout tights for $10 or $15 dollars! Well not totally gone because I have no shame in grabbing some Family Dollar workout tights for the win but, the Family Dollar tights don't give you all the bells and whistles of these new age tights. The new age tights have compression and high waist and other good stuff that makes it almost worth it to catch a sale!

Back to my victory. I had been trying on my size 18 jeans that I bought from Old Navy years ago. I was finally able to get into them, but they fit weird. After several attempts to make my old jeans work, I gave in to a sale Old Navy was having and bought three pairs of jeans. I made the executive decision to size down. I figured, even if I had to wait to get into the size 16 my money would be wisely spent because they will last me a while instead of getting too big too soon.

Much to my surprise and joy I tried on the size 16 jeans, and they fit! It may be the stretch in the jeans, but I don't care! Most jeans are made with a little stretch nowadays. I had absolutely no struggles with pulling, zipping, or buttoning up the jeans! While there is still room for them to fit better, I can also say that they are not uncomfortable! This excites me! My original goal was to get down to a size 14. Can you believe I am only a dress size away from my goal?

At my highest weight I was a size 22. Literally, the last pair of dress pants I bought were a size 22. I had to finally give in, get out of my denial, and get the size 22 pants because the size 20 pants were too tight. That was a low and sad place for me. I could not believe that I had really gotten that big.

The funny part is, I honestly only got to wear those size 22 pants a few times. The pandemic hit which caused me to begin to work from home. Then I started this weight loss journey which had me out of the size 22 in no time.

I see a closet cleaning in the very near future. I have too many clothes anyway. Now would be a good time to go ahead and sort through my too big attire and donate to Goodwill.

You know, I held on to those size 18 jeans for years with the mindset that I would get myself together, lose the weight, and get back into them one day. I don't know if holding on to those jeans all these years held me back in any way, other than taking up space in my closet. What I do know is, there was no point in me holding on to them for so long only to not have use for them.

While they will get donated and hopefully be useful for someone else, it makes me think and reflect on how often we hold on to things that we will never have use for again. We hold on to things thinking they will be good for us later only to find out God wants to replace it with even greater, something shiny and new. Throw them too small clothes away sis! Throw away the baggage bro! God will replace it with even better!

64.2 Pounds down
April 17, 2021

I've hit a plateau. I lost about 10 pounds after my birthday but March and April thus far I have seen no progress. I also have not seen any setbacks either as I have not gained any pounds. I just find myself in this continuous circle of weighing in between 218-220. There were about two weeks in March where I lost momentum exercising and when I picked back up, I didn't hit the exercise hard. I also picked up eating. I did not pick up bad things like dessert! However, I did find myself in a place where I was feeling hungry all the time like when I first started my journey.

The past three weeks I have begun incorporating jogging into my routine. Remember I said I was going to do that? Well, I kept my word, albeit later than expected. The first week of jogs I utilized the back side of my neighborhood to jog and struggle and breathe hard. The first day I was able to run a good stretch and finish walking. The second day, perhaps because I had too much time to think about the task at hand, I really struggled, and my pace was off.

One morning a guy walking his dog in my neighborhood passed by. I said good morning and his response was "oh you are out of breath." I wanted to say, "no shit Sherlock," but I simply said yeah and kept pushing. After week one of my jogging, I had gotten myself in a routine of alternating between walking and jogging. I'd walk the first half of my exercise. Then I would jog a few minutes. Walk a few minutes to catch my breath and then jog some more.

I finally ran into the lady that works closely with the homeowner's association and was able to get the community clubhouse code. This week I decided to try out the treadmill in the community clubhouse. Each morning I walked to the clubhouse. Walked on the treadmill for about 10 minutes, jogged for 10 minutes, walked another 10 and then walked home. On a few days I added a few minutes extra of jogging and less walking on my last walking interval. I hope to increase my time jogging.

I've found that I like the treadmill better. I can set my pace and keep it the same which helps with my breathing and endurance. I plan to keep this routine and prayerfully I will break this plateau and begin losing again. Since my mom is out of town this week, I also plan to go meatless. I've stocked up on my salad fixings, veggies, and plant-based meat options such as veggie sausage, veggie burgers, tofu and chik'n patties. Hopefully, this change in diet will also shock my body into breaking the plateau. I am certainly not finished with this journey yet and hope to see some more results soon.

65.7 Pounds Down

April 22, 2021

The week is not yet over, and I am making progress. I will absolutely take that 1.5-pound loss! Thus far this week I have run three times and walked each day. I have kept it simple with my meals. For breakfast I have done two boiled eggs, two veggie sausage patties, either an orange or yogurt and coffee. For lunch I have done either a green salad (one of those good old throw all the things I like in a salad, eggs, and balsamic vinaigrette) or fruit salad (1 apple, 1 banana, 1-2 mandarin oranges). Some of the mornings I have also opted for the fruit salad instead.

My dinners have varied from a green salad, veggie burger, tofu teriyaki veggie stir fry to a 12-piece Chick-fil-A nugget and fries. Look, I was out and about too long on Wednesday, and it was either eat or die! No but seriously, I resisted getting a sandwich to cut out the bread and I did not get a chocolate chip cookie. That was a win in my book! I will continue with no meat for the remainder of the week and plan accordingly.

I made a discovery that gave me a boost of encouragement this week. I went in to check my heart rate on my Fitbit app. One of the things that the Fitbit measures is cardio fitness. To my surprise, I have moved from the poor cardio fitness level to the average cardio fitness level for women in my age range. I remember at the beginning of my journey being at the very low range of the poor cardio fitness level. This is an achievement I am proud of. I will continue in hopes of meeting the good, very good and excellent ranges.

I can feel the improvement in my body with my jogging. I have found that generally once I have jogged for about 10 minutes, as the saints would say, I feel my help coming on! I have a desire to press and jog longer. I think this is called like a runner's high or something to that effect. I am enjoying the fact that my body desires more movement, and I will continue to press and challenge myself to move.

67.3 Pounds Down

May 4, 2021

I weighed in at 215.6 pounds. I am so happy to see 215, you just do not know! I am not going to lie, since my last weigh in I have binged and ate Bojangles for several meals. Their biscuits never tasted better! In addition to Bojangles, yes, I did something that I have not done in almost a year and that is order a Domino's pizza. It was the thin crust, so I do not feel bad.

I also found myself binging on these random brownie crisps that I found in Dollar General. I wanted a snack and needed to find a healthy option but did not. The blonde brownies were reminiscent of my grandmother Dof's friend Aunie's sugar cookies. It took me back a bit! It is funny how food just takes you back to memories and comfort places.

How is it that I continue to lose weight when I have binged on crazy things? I would say that I have remained consistent in my exercise. What I am also realizing is that I am probably not eating enough. Perhaps my body had gone into starvation mode, and I needed a little binge for my body to release the fat it was trying to hold on to.

Over the next few weeks, I will be working on increasing my food intake in a healthy way. I am considering very hard the keto diet, or at least increasing my protein and lowering my carb intakes.

In terms of my exercise, in addition to my jogging, I also need to make use of the weights that I have purchased. I have a set of three-pound and five-pound dumbbells as well as an up to 12-pound adjustable kettle bell. I did a cool kettle bell workout last week that I need to try and incorporate at least two times a week.

It seems like most of my purchases now days revolve around fitness. I bought some Brooks running shoes of which run well but rub the heck out of the back of my ankles. One day I decided I would put band aids on my ankles to try and protect them. When I got home, I had drawn blood so to Amazon I went and ordered some running ankle socks.

Who would have thought that I, Kendra Allenette Wood, would be so dedicated to my fitness that I would draw blood and get battle scars? I would have never imagined. The running socks worked perfectly. This was such a relief not only in terms of the pain but also my pockets because Brooks are not cheap!

71.3 Pounds Down

May 14, 2021

Don't stop short of the blessing! Last week I was on the treadmill. I was struggling a little bit and it dropped into my spirit, "Don't stop short of the blessing!" That word kept me jogging through to my goal during that exercise session. That word has also continued to pop up every so often over the past week.

I found that this is perhaps my mantra for the last leg of my journey. When I was in my plateau, I started thinking oh, maybe if I can just get under 200 pounds, I'll be happy with that. I don't need to get down to 180 as long as I can get under 200 pounds. But I kept at my exercise and am seeing my weight loss begin again and I will not stop short of my blessing. I will not stop short of my goal.

My current weight is 211.6 pounds. I only have 31.6 pounds to go to reach 180 pounds. I am hoping that I can get under 200 pounds by the end of June. My plan is to continue what I have been doing. I've learned on my journey that my consistency is what has paid off the most.

When I mention "my consistency" I really have to back that up to say my God led, God kept, God motivated consistency. It's funny, I saw a post online that addressed the whole concept of "manifesting." It has become a popular yet ill-informed trend for folks to say they are manifesting their dreams, goals, and vision.

I've never subscribed to that concept. I've always known my source to be God. I trust God to bring to fruition, make manifest, the promises he has for me. He promises me a hope and a future, according to Jeremiah 29:11. I can't have a hope and a future without my health. He also promises me that by his stripes I am healed (Isaiah 53:5). I trust him to keep his promise to heal me of obesity, food addiction, hypertension, and the emotional and mental stressors that would cause me to eat an unhealthy way.

I can't manifest a doggone thing, but I know a man who does not withhold good things from his children (Luke 12:32). Where I am weak, he is strong (2 Corinthians 12:9-11). Where I want the cake, he gives me the restraint to walk away and drink some water instead. Where I want to sleep in and not get in this morning workout, he wakes me up and blesses me with the motivation and ability to move.

I can take no credit for this 71.3-pound weight loss. It is the God in me that has allowed me to see this and will allow me to see it through to my goal of 100-pound weight loss!

73 Pounds Down

May 16, 2021

This morning I weighed in at 209.8 which puts me at exactly 73 pounds down in my weight loss journey. In addition to this scale victory, I was also able to sell about half a closet worth of my too big clothes during a community garage sale that happened in my neighborhood.

As opposed to lugging the remainder of my clothes back upstairs and in my closet, I bagged those items and took them straight to Goodwill. It felt good to purge. Just like I am releasing this weight, I am also releasing the stuff! So often we let the stuff pile up when we really don't need it at all.

Speaking of stuff that we hold on to, I really have to unpack, or better yet bag up and purge some mental stuff, these feelings that I am beginning to have when I look back at my fat pictures and when I make comparison pictures. I get this extreme sadness when I look at my fat pictures. And I am struggling to pinpoint the root of my depression or unhappiness that let me gain so much weight.

I also look at those pictures like why Ya'll let me get this fat? I know, I am pointing the finger. I also can't lie and say that no one said anything to me, because some of my closest friends/family said things, but when you love someone, there is that grace that you give to let them get to where they need to be in their own time. I appreciate that grace. However, from this point on, family and friends, do not let me go back to where I came from! Scream it to the roof tops if you have to!

I am also finding that I need to give myself some grace when it comes to my body image and not allow the enemy to creep in and tell me that I am not skinny enough. I mentioned the struggle with comparison pictures. I've found myself looking at comparison pictures and having a hard time seeing the difference in my fat pictures and my current pictures.

This is a lie! I will not allow myself to view myself through any lens other than the truth. The truth is, I've lost a whole 73 pounds, closer to 80 pounds if I consider my highest weight at some point was 289. I am healthier and feel better than I've felt in a long time. I am fearfully and wonderfully made. I am not defined by a scale.

I intend on guarding my heart and my mind with these truths and any other truths from God as I strive toward losing my last 30 pounds. I pray against seeing anything other than God's truth in the mirror now and once I reach my goal weight.

1.6 Pounds Up

May 25, 2021

Yes, you read that correctly! In fact, somewhere over this past weekend I was 5.2 pounds up weighing in at 215. Could it all be water weight? Absolutely! But I wanted to check in at this 1.6 pounds up to share a few of my secrets.

First things first, this is one of many ups and downs along this journey. In fact, I only really log my weight when I have lost pounds. In my weight loss journey and in your own you will have losses, plateaus, and gains. However, you have got to remain consistent and keep going.

During my plateau I was rethinking my goal, ready to settle with getting to 200 pounds instead of 180. Now while I have made a conscious decision to be at peace if I don't lose another pound, I have also gotten to a point where I refuse to stop short of my blessing and not work to lose this 31.6 pounds. Losing 31.6 pounds is an attainable goal. I have done it twice over! I will lose those pounds if I just stay consistent.

Be encouraged if you've gained weight or have hit a plateau or even if you're losing but not as quickly as you desire. All things come in God's timing not our own. Ultimately, I am so grateful that I am in better health than I was this time last year. It makes me think of the scripture that said about this time next year you will have a son (2 Kings 4:16). From last year to this year, he has birthed in me a desire and commitment to my physical, spiritual, and mental health.

What is it that God has birthed in you since this time last year? What is it that God intends to birth in you about this time next year? I think I can stop and just meditate on that for a moment myself!

Back to 73 Pounds Down

May 26, 2021

And just like that, I weighed back in at 209.8 this morning! This brought me much joy and made me feel my goal to be at or under 200 pounds by the end of June feel attainable. I went a little crazy over the weekend, I am not going to lie. I had fried chicken, Hawaiian rolls, fried oysters, sweet potato fries and ice cream cake! So, I feel my body has just now adjusted and gotten rid of all that bad stuff.

I'm learning now however, that my body weight fluctuates. I could lose a solid three pounds in one week, gain the three back the next week and be back down the three pounds the following week. I do not want to continue in this manner. However, it is also an indicator to me that I need to stop being so glued to the scale. While I like a weekly weigh in, I may need to cut back on my weigh ins.

74.5 Pounds Down

June 1, 2021

Okay, it is a new month, so I had to weigh in. I know I said I may need to stop weighing in so often, but I could not help but get a baseline for the month. I really hope I can drop these 8.3 or nine pounds to get under 200 pounds by the end of this month. It has been kind of hard here in the 210's and under.

The past week or so have also just been hard on the exercise front. I've been tired and just not motivated to get up and out in the mornings. I woke up this morning and got dressed for the gym. When I sat down to put my shoes on, my body was like, 'you can tie these shoes up, but you are going to lay back in the bed.' That is exactly what I did!

I went for a walk later in the day, but I just couldn't get going early this morning. It may have something to do with my menstrual cycle, so I am just trying to give myself a little grace and yet not stop either. I've got goals to reach!

I have the virtual Monument Avenue 10k that I am planning to do at the end of this week. I am looking forward to it. It has been years since I've done it or even had the mindset to do it.

76.5 Pounds Down

June 7, 2021

I weighed in at 206.6 this morning. I hit the 75-pound mark yesterday but really didn't have too much to share. I am proceeding with mainly fish and veggies for the remainder of this month with hopes that I will in fact reach my goal of being 200 or less by the end of the month.

Last week was a bit hit or miss in terms of my exercise, but I think it was because I knew in my head, I would be doing the virtual Monument Avenue 10k over the weekend. I haven't done it since like 2016 or 2017. I got up early on Saturday morning and went for it. Surprisingly, I did not have to do too much weird circling around my neighborhood.

Circling the neighborhood too many times was a concern, especially in the era of Ahmaud Arbery and others who have been gunned down simply minding their business and exercising outside while black. For the most part, my neighborhood is nice, and the people are welcoming. They speak and they wave.

However, I can recall sometime back when my mom and I were walking in a newer undeveloped section of the neighborhood. As we passed a street, there was this truck that just stopped to watch us as we walked. My mom being the old I don't care lady that she is, kindly turned in their direction and waved really hard! We chuckled as we walked along but the incident bothered me. It leaves a lasting bit of anxiety even if minimal.

My experience highlights the anxiety that some Brown and Black people feel when they go out to exercise in their neighborhood or just to do simple things in the world. It's bad enough that we as a people don't move and do active things enough. Having that anxiety to add to the list of not moving does not make things better.

For the virtual 10k I pretty much just walked down every street of my neighborhood and out to the entrances of my neighborhood. This was the first time I've done the 10k and was in shape. I jogged a good eight minutes but walked the remainder of the time. That is an accomplishment.

Saturday afternoon my community had a community cookout and pool party. I met an older gentleman who had the 10k T-shirt on. He and his girlfriend did the 10k on Friday out at Dorey Park in Richmond. He encouraged me to keep it up and even encouraged my mom to get out there and do it.

We had to tell him about that one time she did the 10k and left me in the dust. I looked over and she was on the other side of Monument Avenue waving! That memory will forever stick and motivate me to keep active!

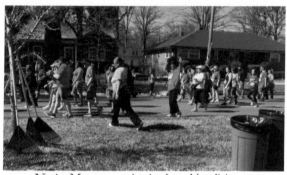

Notice Momma waving in the red hoodie!

3.6 Pounds Up

August 1, 2021

Here we are the first day of August 2021. It's been a while since I stopped to document my journey. Honestly, that is because I've been living my best life during these summer months. I took an impromptu trip to San Diego to visit my cousin that is battling breast cancer. I followed that with a trip to Sarasota to visit my little cousin and enjoy some days at the beach.

I ate what I ate on those trips. I enjoyed chicken and waffles; a variety of carb filled breakfasts. I also enjoyed, ice cream, ice cream, and more ice cream! The following weeks after those trips I never got back into the swing of exercise.

Last week I traveled to Baltimore for my nephew's 16th birthday party and to see my grandma Dof. I have not seen my her since before the pandemic started. On this trip I ate what I ate as well! I enjoyed my time with my family and that is that.

However, it is August. A year ago, this month I made up my mind that I was changing my lifestyle so that I could be in shape and healthy. I did such a great and consistent job from August to January, and it seems I've been struggling a bit ever since.

Despite my struggles, I've made an awesome discovery! My non scale victory is that I am fitting in a size 14 jeans and large tops and dresses! At the beginning of this journey my weight goal was to get down to 180 but my clothing size goal was to get down to a 14. Although I have not hit my 180-pound goal, in fact I'm struggling to break under of 200, I have reached my dress size goal!

I am happy with that. I've said it before but I'm now getting to a place where I am comfortable in my skin, and I would be ok if I did not get any smaller. Would I like to lose more gut? Absolutely, but I have peace with where I am. I'm happy with the woman looking back at me when I look in the mirror.

I am by no means giving up on my 180-pound goal, however, if I do not reach it, I will not be heart broken. Rather than recommitting to a number on the scale, for the anniversary month of my weight loss journey, I am recommitting to a healthy me!

I woke up this morning, talked myself off the ledge about exercising in my neighborhood and did a nice 30 or so minute walk jog. It felt good to get back on my exercise after a two-week hiatus. I'm not stopping now!

76.7 Pounds Down

August 12, 2021

I weighed in this morning at 206.4. I have not been hitting the exercise as hard as I promised myself for the start of August and my one-year anniversary of this journey but hey, it is just that, a journey.

In my prayer and meditation today, I sensed the Lord speaking to my weight loss as a season of preparation. I felt that he was saying to me that he has given me this season of rest, reflection, and restoration of health because the next season he is taking me in to depends on it. This next season of my life, career, and ministry is going to require that I am the best version of myself, physically, mentally, and spiritually.

This makes me hopeful, and it reminds me not to give up on this journey. I must continue to make my health a priority and be ready when God opens the doors to my next season in life. I am looking forward to what he has in store. I can't say that I fully know what is next, but he sure has given me glimmers of what it could be.

This weight loss journey is so much more than the weight itself. It's about being in a space where I can pour into others. I hope what you've read so far has poured into you in some way. I hope what I am saying motivates you to not only prioritize your health but also listen to the voice of God, hear, and be obedient to what he is preparing and calling you to in your life.

77.5 Pounds Down

August 16, 2021

I weighed in at 205.6 this morning. I just want to break 200! My exercise is still off. I just can't seem to get on track, so I am going to adjust my eating approach instead.

Besides a few too many Starbucks banana breads I've been doing good with my eating. However, I think I am going to do my own lazy version of JJ Smith's green smoothie cleanse and see how that works out for me.

I already have a smoothie for breakfast daily. I am going to ramp this up to a smoothie for lunch and let my only whole meal be a healthy lean dinner. Where the lazy part comes in is if I don't quite feel like making a smoothie for lunch, I am going to do like I did today and have a pre-made açai bowl and some unsalted mixed nuts.

I will continue to drink my gallon of water a day and my detox tea. What I am learning during this journey is that there are a bunch of techniques and tools to use to reach one's desired goals. I am going to try this smoothie cleanse technique and see how it turns out!

81.1 Pounds Down

September 16, 2021

After several failed attempts, last week I successfully made it through the modified version of JJ Smith's green smoothie cleanse. I got to the weekend, was out of town, and all that went out the window. My lowest weigh in during those eight days was 198.8! I made it to onderland!

I don't feel so bad for going off the rails with my eating over the weekend because I walked four miles with my cousin She'Nita on both Saturday and Sunday. We followed those walks with more walking down at the National Harbor, shopping, and simply enjoying life.

Today, however, I am weighing in at 202. Which is why I am only noting that I am down 81.1 pounds. I'm semi doing green smoothies Wednesday through Friday of this week, but I have plans for the weekend that include good food and wine!

I'll try another full 10 days when I'm past the weekend and when my mom goes out of town again. I found it to work well when my mom is out of town because then I have no food distractions. For instance, as I type, she's downstairs frying chicken wings!

As for exercise, I may have to take it easy for a short while. I developed a blister on my foot from all the walking I did over the weekend. I am coming to a realization that maybe Brooks are not my running shoe. I've been in the Luck Road Run Shop and tried out some shoes. The salesperson recommended Saucony's. I am sorry but insert Souja Boy Meme right now. Saucony's?

Saucony's were in style for some of my peers back in that 2005-2006 era, but I have never in my life worn Saucony's. To make it worse, those Saucony's looked like orthopedic 100s! I overpronate very badly. Especially in my left foot. I probably need those orthopedic 100s, but my vanity just won't let me do it.

The next best fit was New Balances. I am not that much fonder of New Balances. I never had a pair. In fact, when I think of New Balances, I think of the white pair of New Balances my daddy used to have. That was a step up for him considering the fact that he would wear the no name tennis shoes with the two Velcro straps in a heartbeat!

I digress! After some research online, I have ordered some New Balance Fresh Foam X Vongo V5 running shoes. Hopefully, this will be a better fit than the Brooks. I don't want any more blisters, bloodshed, or delays in exercising when I have the motivation to exercise.

20 Pounds Up

January 1, 2022

It's been a while since I've checked in here. So here I am the first day of 2022 up 20 pounds. I never did restart my journey back in the fall. I was tired. I skipped a few days. Days turned in to weeks. Weeks turned in to months. I tried to jumpstart here and there with no commitment. I'm back and the best I can say is I am taking this thing day by day.

I have determined that my weight loss goal for 2022 is to lose and maintain a loss of a minimum of 30 pounds. When I first fell off, I kept thinking, I just need the energy to exercise. However, I began to realize that the energy I was seeking would only come if I exercised! So, at this point ain't nothing to it but to do it!

My mom pitched in for a small home treadmill as my Christmas present. I am planning to commit at least 30 minutes daily. Despite my hangover for drinking too much wine last night I broke in my treadmill. I was aiming for 30 minutes but pressed on to 36 minutes and two miles.

The first 20 minutes I walked. The treadmill is much smaller than a regular gym sized treadmill, so it took a few tries before I felt comfortable jogging. The last 16 minutes I had enough comfort and balance to jog. I got a good sweat. I'm praying that I don't have any pulled/achy muscles from the adjusted stride needed for the treadmill. I think I will need to start incorporating some stretching exercises to avoid any injuries. Yes, I know. I probably should have been stretching all along but hey I'll start now.

15.6 Pounds Up

January 21, 2022

This morning I weighed in a 217.6. I just could never get back into my routine last fall. The holidays came and I ate, drank and was merry! It started off as me inching up to about 208. Then I broke 210. From there 215 and before I knew it by the first day of this year, I weighed in at 221.2 pounds.

For the past couple of weeks, I've teetered back and forth between 220 and 218. This morning I finally dropped below 218. I am encouraged by this because I am slowly working to get back into my exercise routine.

While I have not been on my treadmill daily, I have managed to get quite a few workouts in this month. The more time I spend on the treadmill, the more I am getting that drive and energy back to enjoy exercise. I am getting back on track with my water intake as well.

I had a moment, when teetering back and forth in my weight, of doubt about my 30-pound weight loss goal. However, I know this goal is achievable. I also know that this is something that I do not have to rush on myself. I just need to be patient with the process.

Still 15.2 Pounds Up

February 21, 2022

Ok queue the Groundhog Day loop because I feel like I'm starting where I was just at a month ago all over again. However, insert my birthday on January 27, momma's birthday on February 8 another Maryland birthday celebration for my mom and Valentine's Day! I went all the way up to 223! I ate all the things. I halfway exercised and it showed!

However, today I've weighed in at 217.2. On Feb 15 I started the modified version of the 10-day smoothie cleanse. So far, I am down 4.2 pounds. We will see where I weigh in at the end of the cleanse. After losing minimal pounds thus far on the cleanse, I decided to go back to a tried-and-true practice in my exercise routine which is fasted cardio.

As much as I struggle getting out of the bed in the mornings, if I had to reflect on the one thing in my exercise routine that produced the best results it would be those morning fasted cardio workouts. My morning workouts seem to go by faster and are not as hard to get through. They help me to poop!

I love a regular poop first thing in the morning. Workouts in the morning generally work that poop right on out for me! This helps especially when I'm trying to keep a good track of my weigh ins. I like to weigh in after a good poop and before I consume any water or food for the day. I am looking forward to the results of getting back into my morning workout routine.

14.6 Pounds Up

February 24, 2022

This morning I weighed in at 216.6. You know, I weighed in at 216.6 on January 22, so I am still feeling that ground hog day theme again today. However, I am just happy to see the scale going in the right direction.

I know it is not all about the scale but also my physical, mental, and spiritual health. Over the past few weeks, I've had the opportunity to assess my spiritual health. I participated in a small group with my church that focused on sabbath rest. One of the key elements of that group were understanding what sabbath rest truly was.

We focused on breathing. I noticed that for some time, I have not been breathing. I have been holding my breath for the next best or big thing when God simply wants me to rest and spend time with him. I came to this realization during the small group.

One day that I went for a massage. When I got there, I met a new massage therapist. Like many of the other times with other therapists he asked me if I had any problem areas and how he could help. I explained that I just wanted to relax. He mentioned that his specialty was deep tissue massages. I stated that if there were any areas he came across that needed attention, he could focus there but overall, I was there for relaxation. He said he noticed that my right shoulder looked like it needed some work and we proceeded with the massage.

My shoulders must have been a dead giveaway that I was not ok as I described but instead, I was stressed. He worked on my shoulders, arms, neck, and a great full body massage. At the end however, he gave me some advice. "When you find yourself not breathing, you are not there, you are outside of your body. When you realize that, you should get up from what you are doing, go outside and breathe. Take several deep breaths and when you do that you come to yourself. You can be present, not caught in the future, or the past. Just breathe and be present."

That was a whole word to me! I have been caught so much in the future and what my next career step is, that I am stressing out! Yes, I started this book out with a new job, but the world would have you ready to think ahead, as I have been doing for a while now. And God says, "I got this! You just breathe and be present!" In all of this I had to breathe and release the pressure to perform. Maybe you feel pressure to perform in your career, fitness journey, or other area of your life and God is simply saying breathe and be present!

While I have been in a season of plenty as it relates to physical rest, I have been lacking in the spiritual rest of breathing and being in the presence of God. We know that rest is a key factor in the physical aspect of weight loss and well-being. Rest is also important in the spiritual aspect of well-being.

I discovered that what sabbath rest looked like for me was resting in his presence on the treadmill, walking or jogging in general. Surprisingly enough, one of the exercises around paying attention to my breathing made me realize that I was spending sweet time with God on the treadmill. At first, I was simply thanking God for allowing me to get through a jog without struggling to breathe and passing out, but then the thanks turned in to thanks for other aspects of my life and even hearing God's voice. Hearing God's encouragement of "Don't Stop Short of the Blessing" that day on the treadmill is how the title of this book came about.

I got to the point where I was also viewing my morning time on the treadmill as my first fruits sacrifice of the day for my body and physical movement. I am on a journey to get back to that sabbath rest on the treadmill. It makes sense, especially on this journey. I am coming to embrace another truth that rest is trusting Jesus and what he promised. So, I am trusting him not only for the physical journey but the spiritual journey as well.

Haven't Weighed In

March 13, 2022

I did not weigh in today. I have not weighed in over several weeks. The latest attempt at the green smoothie cleanse was a miss and I have come to a place where I really need to step back and reassess my why?

Part of my why is that I want to live! I want to feel and be healthy. I also want to be healthy enough so that when and if the time comes, I can bear children, have healthy pregnancies, and live to see my children and even grandchildren grow up.

I also must circle back to the fact that in the height of this journey, the Lord was impressing upon me the need to be fit physically, emotionally, spiritually, and mentally to be equipped for this next season of my life. Yes, I just spoke on being in the present and breathing but I also acknowledge that God is preparing me for great responsibility in various areas of my life.

I have recently been reflecting on where this book ends. I realize that this is a lifestyle change and that my story never ends. However, I am beginning to sense an urgency to tell my story. I was recently highlighted by a non-profit owned by two of my friends for women's history month and part of the highlight was a listing of the various roles/titles I have. When I listed author, people were surprised!

While I never did a bunch of promotion, in 2011 I published a book of poetry called "Out of the Heart Flows." It was before the social media of today, so I get why some folks were surprised when I mentioned that I was an author. When I wrote that book of poetry, I was on a journey of discovering my identity and healing after the loss of my dad in 2009, Grandma Irma and Aunt Audrey in 2010.

I've found in this weight loss journey that even still; I am continuing to heal from that loss and the hurts of my childhood. It is funny, I was losing weight in such a consistent manner earlier on in my journey I thought, yeah, I'll drop 100 pounds, publish my book, and use the book to hold me accountable to keep the weight off.

However, in life's true fashion, this journey is not linear. It is a continued choice to start over and over again. I am thankful that I can reflect and perhaps I am at a point in my weight loss journey where I need to ask the Lord to reveal to me what it is that he wants to work on and heal in me that is causing my journey to feel like it is stalling?

Or perhaps I am right where I should be in this leg of the journey. We too often get focused on the end goal that we do not give ourselves the grace we need to just be. While I am not saying give up all together, God's grace is sufficient.

The Reset

May 9, 2022

God's grace is sufficient; however, I have been in a bit of denial about my weight gain. As of today, I have gained about 26 pounds and weigh 224.8 pounds

I knew that I could not leave this journey to chance, so I decided what I need to do most was to seek God, plan, and submit my plans to Him. I just finished a bible reading plan that discussed planning for the weight loss. It was centered around the SMART Goals. SMART Goals are Specific, Measurable, Attainable, Realistic and Time Bound.

Throughout that plan I felt the Lord saying to me, "Write the vision. Make it plain...It will surely come and not delay" Habakkuk 2:2-3. Starting today I will recommit to healthy diet and exercise with a goal of losing 36 pounds by September 9 and maintaining through my birthday January 27 and thereafter.

The bible reading plan advised for me to seek God in my ideal weight. I had not done that before but the goal weight that I had in my mind was 189. I prayed that God would confirm that number or tell me otherwise. This morning I finally decided to do an official weigh in and reset my weight loss goal on my Fitbit. As soon as I opened the weight goal in my Fitbit it was set to 189 and that was my confirmation!

Strategies for meeting my goal are to exercise 3-5 days per week for 30 minutes or more. Drink a gallon of fluids daily (water, tea, coffee). Track my food intake on my Fitbit. Practice and leverage intermittent fasting. Each day spend time with God and choose the healthy choice spiritually and physically.

A Chance to Tell my Story

May 10, 2022

Today I had the opportunity to tell my story about my weight loss journey. One of the ministers from my church has a health and wellness group on Facebook. I was able to join a zoom session and tell my story of how I lost over 80 pounds.

Being able to speak to this group was so refreshing. It was confirmation that I have a story to tell. It was also confirmation for me to not stop short of the blessing!

There were other speakers on the zoom that talked through their journey to weight loss. What I found was that we all had much in common. I hope this book helps you to see how much we have in common and encourages you to stay on your journey. While I have not yet met the shiny goal of losing 100 pounds, I intend to choose every day to do something that will get me closer to that goal.

A few Words in Parting

If I had some parting words, I'd tell you to keep a journal. This book is my journal! Being able to document my journey and process my feelings, thoughts, and revelations along the way have been therapeutic. I love being able to look back through my journals to see how far I've come or to see answered prayers!

This journey is not just physical. We have to sit with the issues of life that cause us to live an unhealthy lifestyle. One of my favorite things about journaling is often I hear from God and can document what he says about me when I am grappling with what I or others may think of me. When we sit with it, release it to God, and hear from God we create space to be healed.

I would also encourage you not to idolize the journey. While you may have goals, you may find out that the original goal you set for yourself was or was not the goal you needed. I found out quickly that a size 14 comes well before 180 pounds. I was able and still can fit a size 14 at 200 plus pounds.

Get to a place where you feel good in your own skin. Before I lost this weight, I found myself lacking the confidence that I thought I would always have. I did not like the woman I saw in the mirror. I was chronically tired. I also suffered with what I would consider a form of anxiety when I would lay down to sleep at night. I had struggles breathing, found myself wheezing and feared I may stop breathing in my sleep and not wake in the morning.

I no longer have these issues. I am confident and comfortable in the skin that I am in. I am not pencil thin or toned but I feel good. I feel better than I've felt in a long time, and I have learned to listen to my body.

Stay on the journey! 1 Corinthians 9:24-27 says, *"Do you not know that in a race all the runners run, but only one gets the prize? Run in such a way as to get the prize. Everyone who competes in the games goes into strict training. They do it to get a crown that will not last, but we do it to get a crown that will last forever. Therefore, I do not run like someone running aimlessly; I do not fight like a boxer beating the air. No, I strike a blow to my body and make it my slave so that after I have preached to*

others, I myself will not be disqualified for the prize."
I believe, with your eyes on the prize and
with a goal of not stopping short of the
blessing, you'll find that the journey is more
about what you gain or release along the way
then the way then the actual destination.
What you gain or release along the way, the
healing and discipline to run the race, will
bring you the prize!

My Journey in Pictures

What is a good weight loss story without pictures? I wanted to share a few pictures of myself from over the years that document my weight. While some of the pictures are regular day to day pictures, others are at major milestones in my life such as graduations, birthdays, and world travels. Take pictures of your journey. Take pictures before you even start. You'll be surprised how far you've come. I know I am!

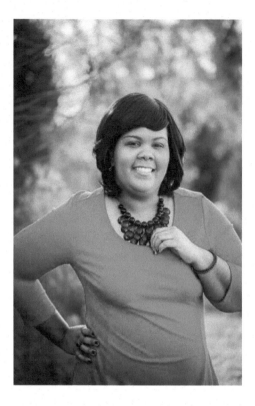

2014: *This photo is from my master's cap and gown/mother daughter photo shoot in November. Around this time, I weighed about 243 pounds.*

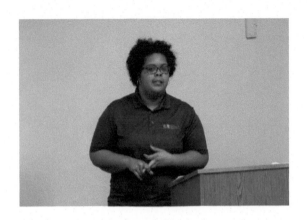

2015: *This picture is from August of 2015. I was leading a new student orientation session at my job. I weighed around 260 pounds.*

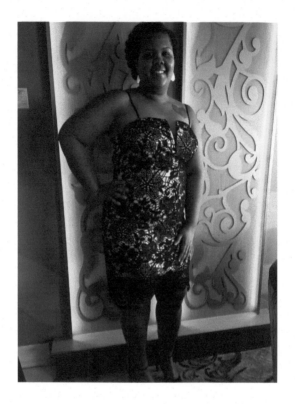

2016: This picture is from September of this year. This is the dress on the cruise to Bermuda where I wore both my girdle and my best friend Dinecia's girdle! I weighed about 249 pounds.

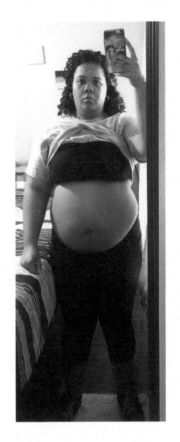

2017: This photo is from June of this year. This was one of my start photos for a weight loss and nutrition program I signed up for. I weighed about 256 pounds here.

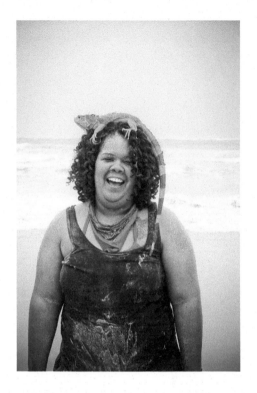

2018: This is from January of this year. I was on my 30th birthday trip to the Dominican Republic. I weighed about 281 pounds here.

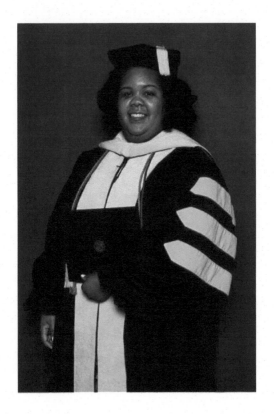

2019: *This is my cap and gown picture from August of this year. I weighed my highest around 289 pounds.*

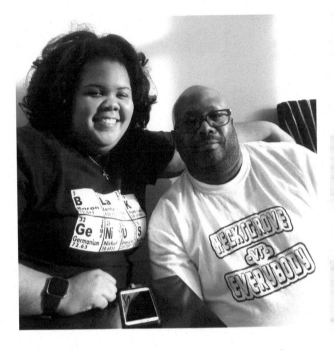

2020: *This was my motivation picture for this journey! My brother Keith had already lost 30-40 pounds in this picture! I weighed around 279 pounds.*

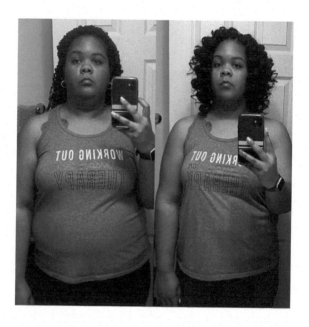

2021: *These are side by sides from September 2020 to January 2021. These pictures were in celebration of 50 pounds weight loss.*

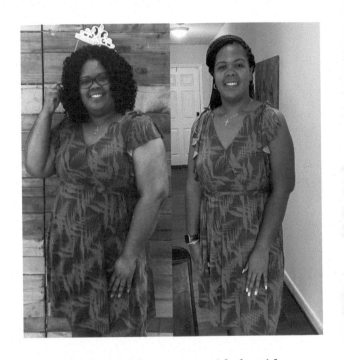

2021: *I had to add one more side by side from 2021. The after photo was in August 2021 for my celebration of 80 pounds weight loss. The before photo is from my cousin's wedding in summer 2018.*

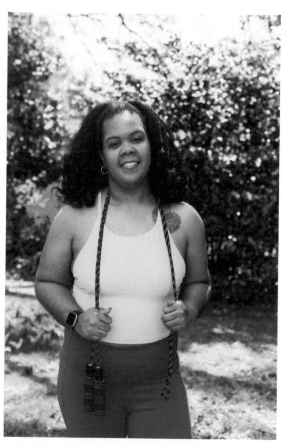

2022: This picture was taken in April. I am not going to lie. I am about 220 in this picture, but I feel good, and I am ready to tackle this forever journey once again!

About the Author

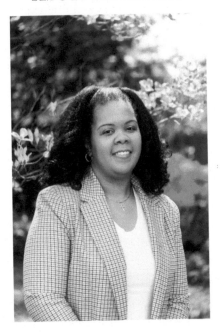

Kendra Wood is a native of and currently resides in Virginia. Kendra spent her childhood and early adult years in Warren County, North Carolina.

She holds a Bachelor of Art in Mass Communication from North Carolina Central University, a Master of Science in Higher Education and a Doctor of

Education in Educational Leadership and Management from Capella University.

Kendra holds over a decade of experience supporting student success in higher education through student services and teaching. While Kendra's career is in higher education, she has found a passion in health and wellness through her fitness journey. Kendra believes in being a lifetime learner and has enjoyed what she has learned on this journey to health and wellness.

Kendra is active in her church and believes wholeheartedly that God sees and cares about his children. She hopes that this book ministers to those on similar journeys. She hopes this book helps others to sit with God in their journey and commit to wholeness physically, mentally, spiritually, and emotionally.

In her free time Kendra enjoys travelling and spending time with her family. Join the virtual fitness community by following Kendra on Instagram @dr.kfit.